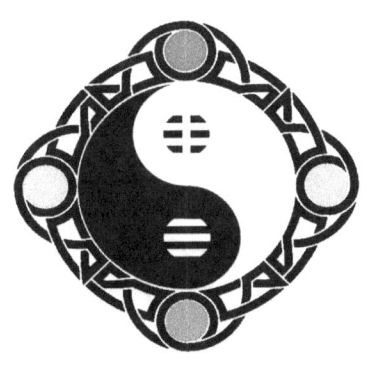

Chi Baton

Exercises

TM ©

By Barry Westley

Published by Barnaby Jay Publications

Main photographs by **Kevin Laidler**.

Supplementary photographs by Stan Griffiths and Ted Parkins.

Testimonials

"Prevention is better than cure!" It is my firm belief that doing these exercises regularly can help prevent and relieve the symptoms of depression, anxiety and M.S., as well as strengthening the body, boosting the immune system and improving the quality of life.

Dr Xiao S F   (Acupuncturist, Herbalist, Tai Chi Practitioner. Kidderminster)

*

Before meeting Barry, I suffered from arthritis of most of my joints; my feet, hands, hips etc. I met Barry through a mutual friend who told me of the Chi Baton™. I was under consultants, hospital appointments, regular physio, the lot. After starting the Chi Baton™ exercises I began to feel better over a period of time. Now I have started back to work and resumed keeping fit again, which I did a lot of before my illness. Since doing Chi Baton™ exercises, I feel my health has improved one hundred per cent. Thank you to Barry.

Steve R (Walsall, West Midlands.)

*

Pure Genius:
Barry Westley and the Chi Baton ™ programmes he has developed.

Wonderful for total body awareness:
- *Breathing techniques.*
- *Energy Movement.*

- *Posture.*
- *Focus Meditation.*
- *Flexibility.*
- *Strength.*

It's part of my daily life.

Lois S.
*

I really enjoy doing these exercises and think they are especially valuable for beginners, as holding the baton ensures that even inexperienced students can easily maintain good posture throughout.

Steve C (Martial Arts instructor, Stourbridge)

*

"After many years of severe back pain and having tried various treatments I was depressed and felt that the pain ruled my life. I came to Barry's class and it completely rebalanced and strengthened my back. With grateful thanks."

Amanda J (Stourbridge, West Midlands.)

This book is dedicated to:

My wife, Louise (for her endless loving support).

Graham Hodgson, (without who's technical help this book would not be completed).

My masters, friends, and students, (living and

dead), and all who daily struggle to perfect their arts.

Contents

Chi Baton™ *exercises are very safe, but you should always consult your doctor before beginning any new exercise regime! If you have any doubts about the suitability of any of the exercises for you, you **must** refer back to your doctor or medical practitioner before attempting them!*

Do not do these exercises if you have been advised against them by your medical practitioner!

Follow the instructions carefully and do not rush, or "bounce", when performing any movement, or part of any movement!

*Do the exercises at a pace that is comfortable for you and only do the number of repetitions that you can **easily** handle. Build up slowly. You should feel refreshed after each of the programmes, not sore and exhausted! Be patient and you will progress more quickly!*

If you feel pain, when performing one of the movements, stop exercising and consult your doctor immediately!

It is also wise to wait at least six weeks before starting, or re-commencing, exercise after giving birth.

Introduction

Welcome to *Chi Baton* ™ .

Chi Baton™ **Exercises,** (formerly known as *Tai Rod Yoga*™ , and *Tai Rod Exercise System*™) is a series of special exercises which are performed using a short rod and are unique to me, **Barry Westley***.

Drawing on my extensive knowledge of Taoist Yoga, Tai Chi Ch'uan, Powerlifting, and a number of different martial arts, (both "hard" and "soft"), I have fashioned an extensive programme of low-impact, rhythmic exercises that strengthen the physical and energetic structure of the body.

Originally devised as a way of teaching principles of body mechanics in a simplified way to my students, *Chi Baton*™ exercises proved to be popular, great fun and surprisingly effective in building internal energy, strength, stamina and flexibility.

Although, *Chi Baton*™ programmes were originally intended for myself and my immediate students, interest in this simple but effective system has grown to such an extent that I felt compelled to write this manual. It can be used on its own or as a compliment to other *Chi Baton*™ videos and DVD's.

A *Chi Baton*™ is a piece of wood twelve and a half inches long which is held between the palms during exercise. (The length is of crucial importance as it gives the correct angles when exercising.)

It may also be made of copper or a mixture of copper

and wood, or plastic and copper.

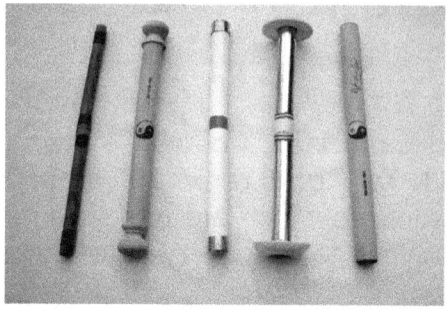

The easiest way to construct a *Chi Baton*™ is simply to cut a piece of doweling the correct length (12 and a half inches, or 318 millimetres, and sand the cut ends.)

A *Chi Baton*™ is not to be confused with a Tai Chi Ruler which is a different length and, to my knowledge, used in quite a different way.

A *Chi Baton*™ can be as simple as the one illustrated, simply a length of dowel, with rounded ends. I like to insert an upholstery tack into the ends to help stimulate

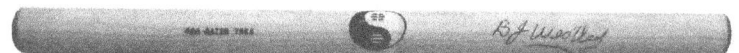

the acupuncture point in the palm of the hand.

Although, this *Chi Baton*™ design is ideal for use with this manual, some students prefer to make their own with varying degrees of complexity.

However, the important principle is that the rod is

comfortable, the correct length, and that you continue to use the same rod each time you exercise. In this way it becomes part of you and infused with your energy, increasing the power of your practice.

(***Barry Westley** has studied **Li Style Tai Chi Chu'an** and **Taoist Yoga** for over 35 years and is a black jacket instructor **(3rd Tengchi)**

He is also a black jacket instructor in **Feng Shou Kung Fu (1st Tengchi),** is a qualified referee in **Tui Shou ("Pushing Hands.")** and **Chinese Martial Forms**, has successfully competed in National Tui Shou Competitions and has represented **England** in the sport of **Powerlifting**.

Barry Westley is also a fully qualified **Shiatsu Practitioner** and **Associate Member of Malvern College of Healing**.)

Basic Principles of Chi Baton™ Exercises

N.B. When learning the exercises do not overload yourself trying to remember all of the principles below, at one time. Learn the exercises thoroughly and gradually introduce each improvement when you feel it is appropriate to you. You will still derive considerable benefit from the exercises even if you forget some of the principles, provided you do not compromise the safe execution of the movements. Always remember, your energy will flow much better when you are relaxed. It is particularly important that you don't let technical considerations spoil your enjoyment of the programmes!

The principles of *Chi Baton™* exercises are similar to those of Tai Chi Ch'uan and Taoist Yoga, ***with some significant variations.*** Although detailed instruction will be given for each exercise, it is wise to keep in mind the following:

1. **Head is held erect** as if being lifted slightly through the crown.

(This can be practiced by placing the tip of the nose against the wall and lengthening the back of the neck without allowing the nose to move.)

2. **Shoulders are relaxed**.

Even when raising arms above the head the shoulders stay down, using the ball and socket joint of the shoulders to effect the movement rather than lifting the shoulders upwards. The simplest way to achieve this effect is to imagine that your hand is resting on a balloon that is gradually inflating and rising up to lift the relaxed arm (i.e. "weight underside"). In this way the correct muscles are used to lift the arm, and the elbows remain soft and without tension.

If both arms are raised at the same time, it is important to look up, allowing the chin to drift forward slightly as you do so, as this relieves the pressure on the blood vessels in the neck.

3. **Joints are never fully locked.**

Even where the arms and legs are straight, the elbows and knees are not fully locked. It should be possible to move easily from one movement to another without having to "release a joint."

4. **Tongue is placed on the roof of the mouth.**

Generally the tongue is placed on the roof of the mouth, just behind the front teeth, during the "expression" phase of a movement. The tongue is dropped from the mouth as the body "releases."

In this way, *Chi Baton*™ exercises differs from many forms of Chinese Yoga and Tai Chi Ch'uan, where the tongue remains on the roof of the mouth at all times.

In *Chi Baton*™, the intention is that the energy pulses as in an "alternating" current electric charge, rather than continuously flowing as in a "direct" current. (It is my personal belief that performing the exercises in this way makes them more dynamic and powerful).

The "expression" may take place in either the in or out breath of a movement, or in some cases, the expression and release may take place during a single breath.

5. Weight is evenly spread over the whole "load bearing" area of the foot.
The weight should feel as if it is evenly spread over the following areas; the heel, outside edge of the foot, both sides of the ball of the foot and the five toes.

(Obviously there will be less weight on the little toe than the heel, but all elements of the foot should feel as if they are equally contributing to the stability of the stance).

6. During the majority of *Chi Baton*™ exercises, movements the waist turns independently of the hips.

This ensures that the feet remain planted firmly and the knees remain in line with the feet. It also ensures that the correct strengthening movement is performed.

When performing the waist twists the hips should remain facing forwards, so that abdomen rotates inside the bowl of the pelvis, rather like a globe revolves in its stand.

Although labelled a "waist twist", the movement should originate deep within the bowl of the pelvis, and spiral upwards through the torso. Generally, the spine should remain straight (Unless, of course, the movement is intended to twist the spine for therapeutic reasons. If the spine twists on normal exercises, the movement is not starting deep enough in the pelvis, the movement is too large, or the shoulder is drawing too far backwards and losing its connection with the turn of the waist.) .

The hips remain forward even when the weight is being transferred to another stance. This helps to prevent the hips drawing out of line or the knees being stressed.

7. The *Chi Baton*™ movements are performed in an even-paced rhythmic manner.

Although there is some flexibility in the actual speed of performing the movements, once that speed is decided upon it must be maintained throughout the programme.

That is, there should be no speeding up or slowing down, when performing an individual movement. In this way the maximum strengthening effect is safely produced with the minimum effort.

Ideally the *Chi Baton*™ should be <u>continually moving, without pauses</u>. (For example, where a movement involves the arms extending outwards and then drawing inwards, it is best to put in a tiny loop at the extreme of each movement to ensure that the *Chi Baton*™ continues to move at all times and that there is not a pause when the baton changes direction).

Generally, in my *Chi Baton*™ classes, the movements are timed to a metronome set at 60 beats per minute. Each movement usually taking four beats. If you do not possess a metronome simply counting the beats "one and two and three...etc.") is perfectly adequate.

Programmes can also be performed at a livelier pace (roughly 72 beats per minute), for a more cardio vascular workout, or at a rhythmic pace to suit you. The important principle is that the exercises are not performed too quickly and that the movements do not speed up or slow down. It is important to resist this temptation as it will impair progress.

8. **Perform the exercises in the order they are given.**

This is important, as many of the exercises act as a "warm up" for the next exercise or as a counterbalance, or "cooling down" for a previous one. It is also important to complete the whole programme, so do not exhaust yourself on the earlier ones so that you can not complete all the units.

If you do not have time to do the whole programme in one sitting, do the standing exercises first, and the sitting exercises later in the day. However, in this case, before commencing the sitting exercises, always perform the first two exercises of the standing programme as a warm up.

9. **Express and Release during each exercise.**

The *expression* can come on either the **in**, or **out** breath, depending on the exercise.

During the *expression* phase one or more of the following should be present. (In an ideal world, of course, the student should perform all simultaneously.):

a)   There is a gradual slight gripping of the toes, causing the instep to rise slightly, and stimulate the kidney 1 ("bubbling springs") acupuncture point in the foot. The best way to perform this is to try to raise the instep slightly, and spread the bones of the feet sideways. In this way, the toes will grip naturally and not "over claw".

(Obviously, it is not appropriate to grip the toes if you are performing certain actions, such as raising your heels.)

b) Gradually and gently contract the anal sphincter.

c) Stretch the spine gently, gradually upwards to the crown of the head.

(Before stretching the spine upwards focus again on "sitting on your dragon's tail" (that is, gently curl the pelvis under as if perching on a shooting stick, and allow the lower back to relax and the knees to flex naturally. When you are competent at this, try to perform the same action just by relaxing the lower back and allowing the pelvis to tilt under). This will allow the upwards stretch to be performed more easily.

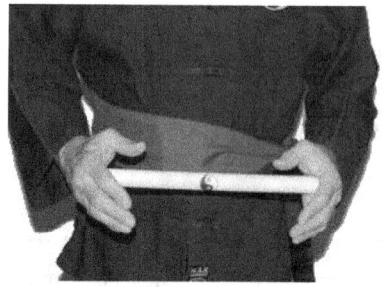

d) Normally the hands are relaxed as if holding a football, with the fingers gently touching and the thumb at a forty-five degree angle.

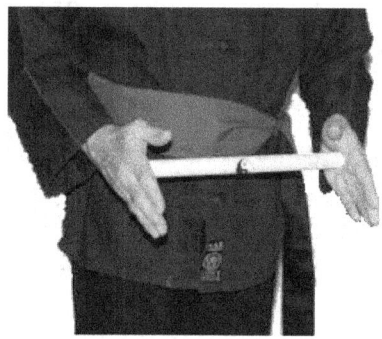

During the **expression** phase of a movement the fingers gently lengthen as if holding a slightly curved box. At the same time the thumb draws back until it is almost in line with the hand, and the bones of the hand are opened sideways. This should slightly increase the pressure at the end of the **Chi Baton**™ and activate the energy centre in the palm. (For this reason, **Chi Batons**™ of my design have a small stud in each end, to improve this contact.) Another way to achieve this expression in the hands is to imagine your hands are partly inflated balloons that further inflate, expand and lengthen during the **expression** phase.

e) The tongue gently contacts the roof of the mouth, just behind the teeth at the start of the **expression** phase.

During the **release** phase, everything gradually returns to the fully relaxed, start position, with the tongue no longer on the roof of the mouth. .

N.B. *There is a lot to learn when* **expressing** *and* **releasing.** *You do not have to remember all the points immediately. Learn the basic movements, thoroughly, and then add an extra subtlety at regular intervals, to maintain your interest and improve your technique.*

10. Breathe in through the nose and out through the mouth.

Breathe naturally in to the belly, the movement of the **Chi Baton**™ will direct the breath where it needs to be.

Remember that sometimes the exercise will make the breathing easier to perform (as for a Buddhist breath) and at other times the exercise will seem to make breathing more difficult (as for a Taoist compression breath). Both types of exercise are equally valid.

In some exercises both types of breathing are present.

11. In general, keep weight "underside".

When raising and lowering any part of the body while performing a movement of the **Chi Baton**™, direct your attention to the underside (that is, the side nearest the ground.)

This will produce a heavy sensation in the limb or body so that the action is both more relaxed and yet slightly more challenging. One way of understanding "weight underside" is to imagine that a balloon is inflating under the part of the body to be lifted. When lowering that part of the body imagine it is resting on a slowly deflating balloon.

Doing the exercises in this way has a more profound effect on the body's energy system and so you may feel tired for a while after exercising, until your body becomes accustomed to it.

N.B. Although it is not within the scope of this manual, it is a very good idea to "stretch out" after every workout programme.

Although, almost every movement in *Chi Baton*™ contains a large element of stretching, spending a few extra minutes on held (but not forced), medium range, stretches will pay dividends, helping prevent excess lactic acid build up in the muscles.

The Chi Baton © Logo

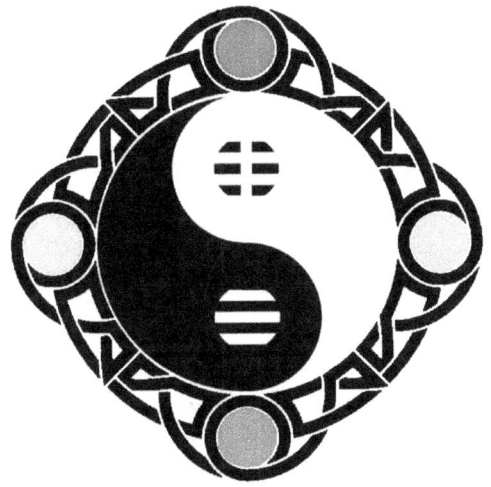

In developing the **Chi Baton**™ system of exercises I decided to design and adopt a specific Logo that reflected the spirit and aims of these exercises.

As the bulk of the exercises were based on the the Taoist system of Chinese Yoga and Chi Kung, I based the logo on the well known Yin and Yang symbol. To this, my good friend Chris Van Dyke added the knot-work representing the movement of the Tao, five elements and much more sacred symbolism.

To further emphasise the spiritual aspect of this work, I cast the I Ching and came up with the hexagram T'ai.

This struck me as particularly relevant, not least because of the strong links **Chi Baton**™ has with T'ai Chi Ch'uan.

I decided to combine these to symbols to create, what I feel, is a logo of profound meaning and deep spiritual power.

In the logo, as in the I Ching, T'ai is for Peace, Harmony and Benevolence. With the trigram for earth (three black broken yin lines) being placed over the trigram for sky (three unbroken white yang lines). The sky intermingles with the earth. This is a very fortunate symbol. (Literally, "Heaven on Earth")

It is also about the strong supporting the weak, doing the right thing at the right time, and small offerings bringing large rewards. ("Less is more" to paraphrase the great Taoist book "The Tao Te Ching").It is about the strong and rigid force creating harmony with the weaker by being flexible and yielding.

The exercises within this book were devised through intense study, together with meditation, dowsing and channeling, so a spiritual thread runs through them all. It is my personal belief that regular practice of these exercises can benefit an individual on the mental and spiritual levels as well as on the purely physical. I hope, in time, you will feel able to agree.

Chi Baton™ Programmes

This manual contains the first **Chi Baton**™ programme.

Although this programme is entire unto itself, there are, at present, a further 40, hour long exercise programmes taught within the system, which have been pioneered, and developed, in my exercise classes over the past fifteen years. Should this book prove successful, I hope to disseminate more information through a variety of media in the future.

Each of the **Chi Baton**™ programmes is put together for a different purpose and, although each programme is complete and stands on its own, the ideal is to rotate between them all. (This ensures that you do not become bored and that the body is being continually challenged to stimulate it to grow.) A few exercises will re-appear in different programmes. This is because I am convinced of their particular value.

Each exercise will contain a **suggested** number of repetitions, but obviously the student can perform more or less repetitions. The important thing is that you do not overtax yourself! (You should feel refreshed, not exhausted at the end of the session). Aim to perform a roughly equal amount of repetitions for each exercise so that the programme retains its balance.

This first programme introduces the basic principles of **Chi Baton**™. It is formulated to improve the cardio-vascular system, balance and posture, stretch all the major muscle groups, teach correct breathing, and improve the flow of internal energy (chi) by "opening the gates" of the body. It also emphasises using the body's natural planes of movement, and encourages using the muscles and joints in a harmonious fashion.

Chi Baton™ Stances

Chi Baton™ stances are based on those of the *Li (Lee) Family Style of Tai Chi and Taoist Yoga.* (The Li Style is, historically, an offshoot of the Wu Style). <u>Remember, when performing the stances that the knees are hinge joints and should always point in the same direction as the middle toes of the feet.</u>

Where indicated, the *Chi Baton™* can be used as a useful tool to aid measurement of these stances.

<u>*Eagle Stance*</u>

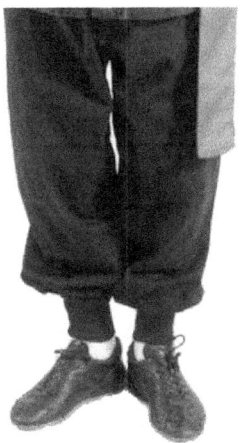

Stand with heels touching and feet at a natural angle. The weight is evenly spread over the soles of the feet with the toes in contact with the ground.

The knees and hips are relaxed as if "sitting on a dragon's tail" (or "perching on a bar stool", if that is an image closer to home!).

The spine and head are held erect as if the head is being suspended from a thread. (Be careful to extend through the rear of the neck and not to push the chin forwards!)

The shoulder blades are open and the shoulders relaxed.

There is always a space between the arms and the body.

The hands are slightly curved with the fingers either touching or very close together. The thumb is at an angle roughly 45 degrees from the hand.

The tongue is gently touching the roof of the mouth just behind the front teeth.

Bear Stance

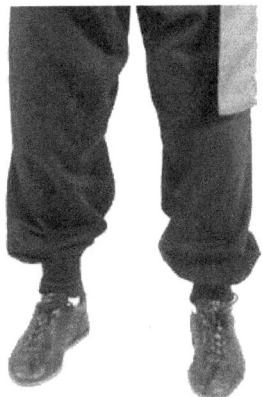

The feet are parallel to each other, roughly one **Chi Baton**™ distance apart, from the centre of each foot.

To check your stance hold the **Chi Baton**™ between the palms with the fingers straight, bend forward. Your finger tips should touch the centre of each foot.

To perform the stance, imagine "sitting on your dragon's tail". That is, slightly curve the pelvis under and allow the knees to gently bend to compensate for this action. Do not over bend the knees, as this will weaken the posture.

(N.B. The purpose of slightly curving the pelvis under is to flatten out the hollow of the back. In a perfect world, the hollow of the back would be flattened to allow the pelvis to sink, rather than the other way round, but as it is easier to perform the first action it is probably wise to master this and feel what the action feels like before trying to reproduce it the second way.)

The rest of the posture is the same as for eagle stance.

Goat Riding Stance

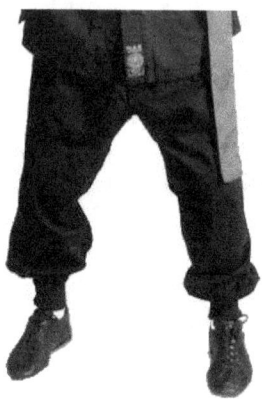

This is the same as for *bear stance* except that the feet are one and a half **Chi Baton**™ distances apart.

As for *bear stance,* "sit on your dragon's tail", to slightly curve the pelvis under and allow the knees to gently bend. (Remember not to over bend the knees!)

Goat riding stance is not traditionally used in the Li Style Tai Chi, but I have included it in **Chi Baton**™, as it is a perfect transitional stance.

Horse Riding Stance

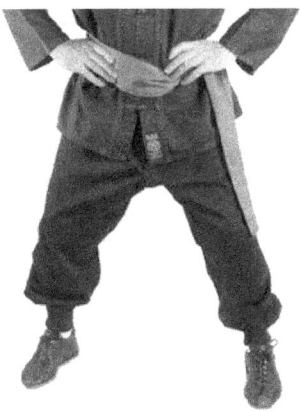

This is the same as for **bear stance** except that the feet are two _Chi Baton_™ distances apart. (Measured from middle toe to middle toe).

As for _bear stance,_ "sit on your dragon's tail", to slightly curve the pelvis under and allow the knees to gently bend. (Remember not to over bend the knees!)

It is particularly important in this stance not to force the knees apart or let them drift inwards. Make sure that the nine points of the feet are in contact with the ground, with the weight evenly spread over the feet, to ensure that the knees are in the correct position.

Leg Triangle Stance

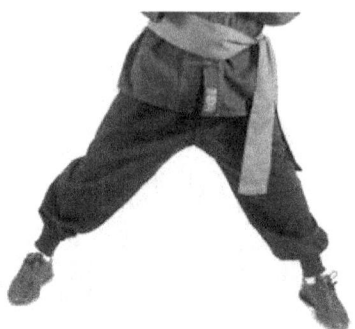

Superficially similar to *horse riding stance*, in this stance, the feet are three **Chi Baton**™ distances apart.

The legs are straight but the knees are not locked.

Although the legs are straight, you should still endeavour to "sit on your dragon's tail", so that the pelvis is slightly tucked under and the lower back flattened somewhat.

(N.B. It is virtually impossible to adequately relax the pelvis if the legs are locked!)

As for the above stances, make sure that the weight is evenly spread over the whole of the feet.

Dragon Stance

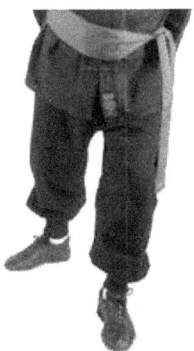

To achieve this stance, step directly forward from eagle. The front leg bent (bearing approximately 70 per cent of the body's weight) and the rear leg straight but not locked (bearing approximately 30 per cent of the body's weight).

The feet are one and a half **Chi Baton**™ distances apart (measuring from middle toe to middle toe) as if standing on two narrow rails.

The front foot faces forward and the rear foot is at a 45 degree angle, with the hips facing forwards.

The front knee acts as a hinge and always faces in the direction of the middle toe. It does not extend beyond the end of the toe at any time.

The spine is lengthened at a natural inclined angle, in line with the back leg. (Do not force the body upright in this stance as it will cause discomfort in the lower back.)

Duck Stance

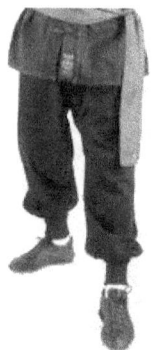

This can be obtained by simply transferring the weight from a **dragon stance** by tucking the pelvis under to transfer the weight to a slightly bent rear leg. The rear leg bears 80 per cent of the weight.

The front foot is flat and the spine erect.

Plough Stance

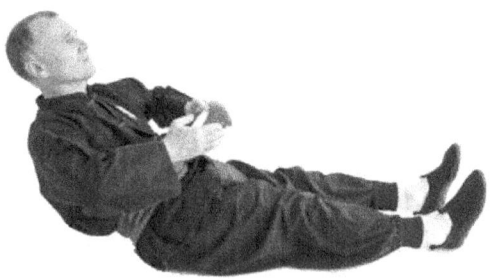

Sit on the floor with the legs outstretched, feet pointing upwards, with the spine and head inclined at a forty-five degree angle.

There should be a space between the feet (approximately one *Chi Baton*™ length from centre toe to centre toe), so that the hips, knees and ankles are all in a straight line.

(In this, and many other *Chi Baton*™ exercises, the elbows are lifted as if by balloons, with the baton in line with the centre of the chest. As you lift the elbows, draw them outwards to ensure that the shoulder blades remain spread) ..

Fish Stance

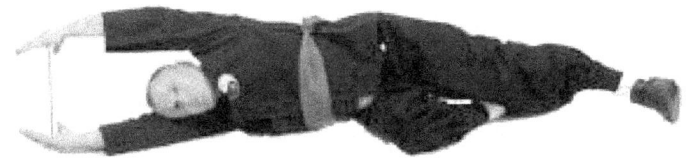

Lie on your right side with the *Chi Baton*™ held above your head, with your head resting on your right arm. This should ensure that the spine is kept straight.

The lower leg is bent with the knee forwards and heel drawn up towards the buttocks at an angle comfortable for you.

Cobra Stance

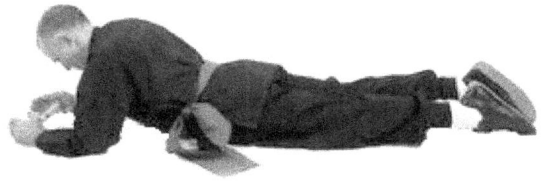

Lie face down on the floor with the **Chi Baton**™ held between the hands and the forearms resting on the floor.

The feet are one **Chi Baton**™ apart, from middle toe to middle toe.

<u>In this position the upper body is raised from the ground. It is important that the front of the hips remain on the floor at all times when in this position to ensure that the back is not strained, and that the weight is distributed evenly over the whole of the forearm, and not just focussed on the elbow.</u>

Crocodile Stance

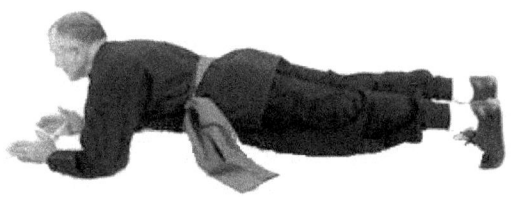

Begin in **cobra stance**, curl toes under, then raise the hips so that the body is now supported by the whole of the forearms and the tips of the toes. The body is held straight and is parallel to the ground.

Chicken Stance

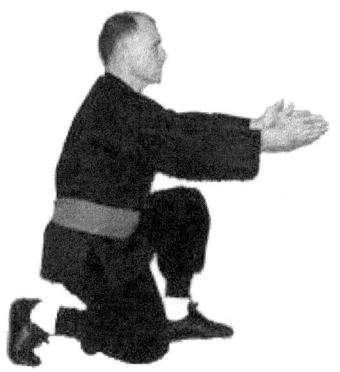

Stand in **goat riding stance**, then turn to the left, rotating on the left heel. Now lower the body, as if sliding down a pole, raising the right heel, so that the right knee finishes just behind the left ankle, an inch or so above the ground. **Do not lean forward in this stance as you will overload the front knee!**

TM ©

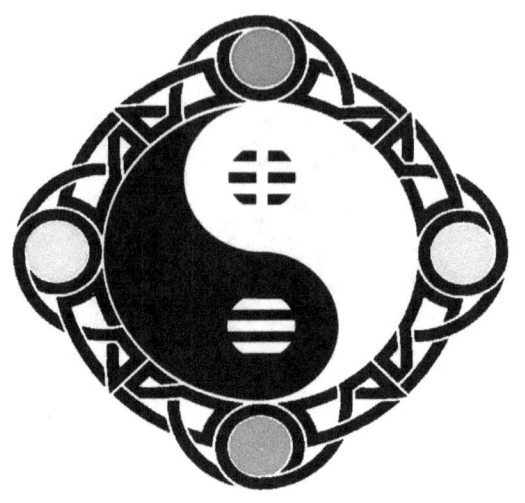

Chi Baton™ ©
Exercise
Programme

Exercise Programme

Stand Still.

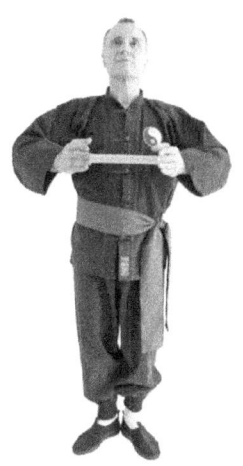

Stand in *Eagle Stance*, holding the rod at chest height, with the shoulders and elbows relaxed. Gently raise the elbows as if they have been lifted by balloons, to form a straight line with the **Chi Baton**™ As you lift the elbows, draw them outwards to ensure that the shoulder blades remain spread Keep the tongue on the roof of the mouth and focus on circulating energy from the heart down the left arm, across the **Chi Baton**™, up the right arm and through the body making a circle.

Do this for about a minute to energise the heart and prepare the body for the work that follows.

Ring the Bell

N.B. Remember! All the movements in the following exercises should be controlled and equally timed. (Approximately four seconds per in breath and four seconds per out breath for a strengthening movement and two to three seconds for a more aerobic workout.)

Start in *eagle* posture, with arms relaxed , and the centre of the **Chi Baton**™ held at one fist distance from the body.

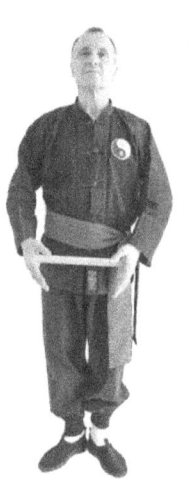
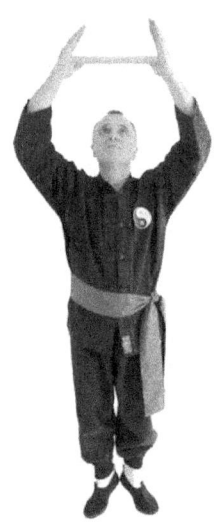

On the in breath, **express**, gradually lifting the arms upwards, being careful not to raise the shoulders. As the **Chi Baton**™ becomes level with your eyes, follow it with your head so that the neck is kept open and free. At the end of the move, draw the elbows outwards, and back slightly, to open up the sides of the chest.

At the same time as you lift the **Chi Baton**™ gradually

raise your heels off the floor as high as you can comfortably manage.

On the out breath, *release*, in a controlled manner, and gradually return to the start position.

Do six repetitions.

N.B. Try to keep your heels touching each other throughout the movements. This helps prevent tipping forward and straining the toes. The knees should relax, and the pelvis tuck under as you make the upward movement, so that the head stays in the same place.

Touch Heaven, Touch Earth

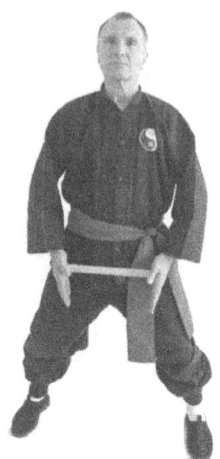

Start in *riding horse* posture, with arms relaxed, fingers pointing down, holding the **Chi Baton** ™ one fist distance from the body.

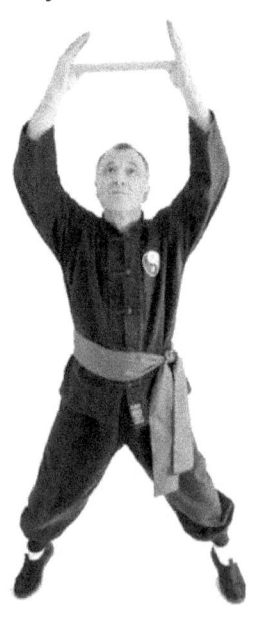

On the in breath, **express**, gradually lifting the arms directly upwards. (Being careful not to raise the shoulders). As the **Chi Baton**™ becomes level with your eyes, follow it with your head so that the neck is kept open and free. At the end of the move, draw the elbows outwards, and back slightly, to open up the sides of the chest.

At the same time as you lift the **Chi Baton**™ gradually raise your heels off the floor as high as you can comfortably manage, and straighten the legs. (But do not lock them).

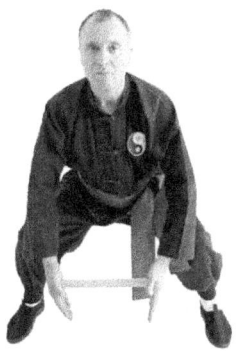

On the out breath, **release**, gradually bending the legs and lowering the heels. When the heels touch the floor continue to squat until your thighs are at least parallel to the ground (i.e. in **deep** *riding horse* stance).

In the next **expression** start from the deep squat position, raising the heels, and straightening the legs, when you reach normal *riding horse* position.

Do six repetitions.

Monkey Dancing

Start in _riding horse_ posture, with arms relaxed, .fingers pointing down, and the centre of the **_Chi Baton_**™ about one fist distance from the body.

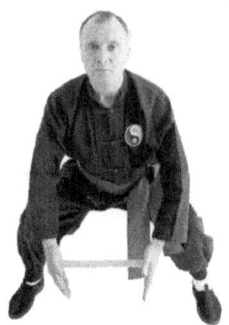

On the out breath, sink into a _deep riding horse_ stance.

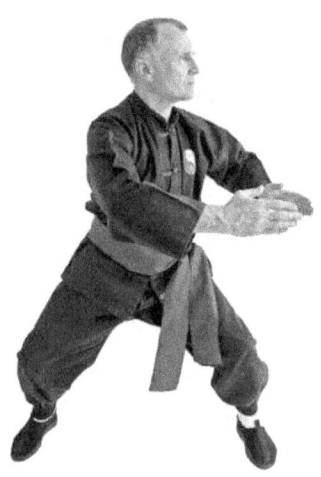

On the in breath, **express** gradually lift the arms upwards and outwards, until they are in line with the centre of your chest. At the same time, twist the waist to the left hand side of your body and rise up into a normal _riding horse_ stance. At the end of the move, lift the elbows and extend them outwards, to open up the sides of the chest.

N.B. Remember the knees do not move in this stance.

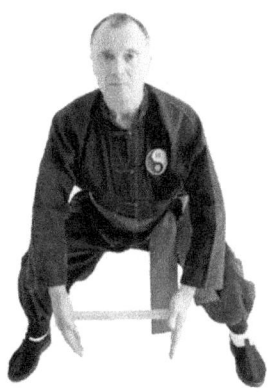

On the out breath, ***release***, in a controlled manner, and sink into a *deep riding horse* stance, lowering your arms and turning to the front as you do so.

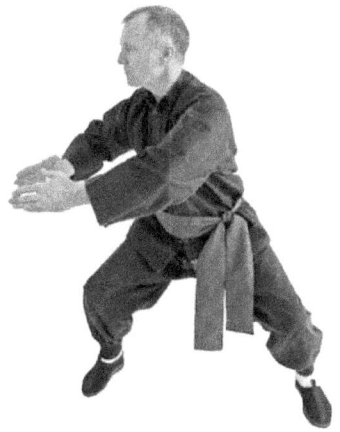

On the in breath, ***express*** gradually lift the arms

upwards until they are in line with the centre of your chest, and twist the waist to the right hand side of your body. At the same time rise up into a normal *riding horse* stance. At the end of the move, lift the elbows and extend them outwards, to open up the sides of the chest.

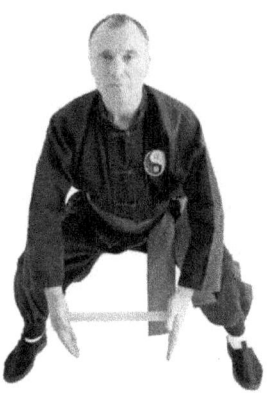

On the out breath, **release**, in a controlled manner, and sink into a *deep riding horse* stance, lowering your arms and turning to the front as you do so.

Do six repetitions each side.

Figure of Eights

(N.B. Keep the centre of the **Chi Baton**™ in line with the centre of your sternum (chest), throughout the exercise).

Start in riding horse posture, with arms relaxed, fingers pointing down and the *Chi Baton*™ one fist distance from the body.

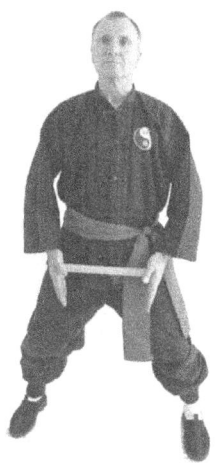

On the in breath, gradually lift the arms upwards until the are in line with the centre of your chest. At the end of the move, lift the elbows and extend them outwards, to open up the sides of the chest. The *Chi Baton*™ is almost two fist distances from the chest.

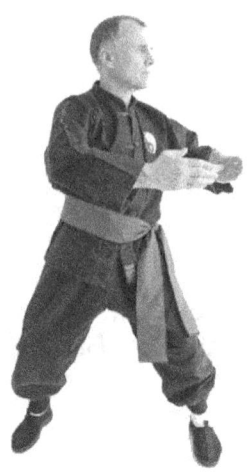

On the out breath, without altering the position of the knees, twist the waist to the left hand side of your body.

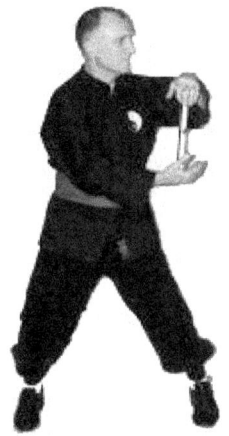

On the in breath, **express,** and rotate the arms clockwise around the centre of the **Chi Baton**™ , so that the left hand is uppermost.

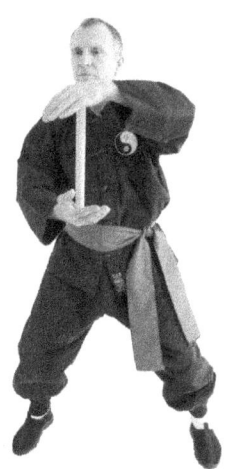

On the out breath, *release,* and twist the waist, through the forward facing position, to the right hand side of your body, keeping the *Chi Baton*™ in the vertical position.

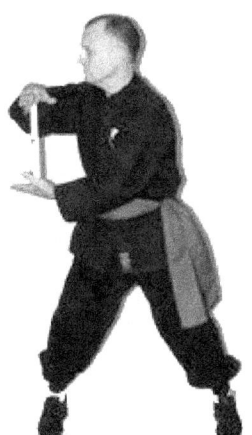

On the in breath, *express,* and rotate the arms anti-clockwise around the centre of the *Chi Baton*™ , so that the right hand is uppermost.

On the out breath, *release,* and twist the waist to the

left hand side of your body etc.

Do six repetitions each side, then, on the final out breath, turn to the front, lowering your arms as you do so.

Disperse the Hornets

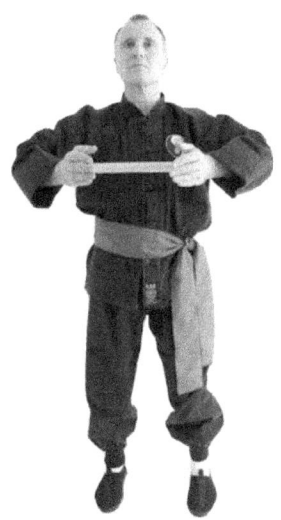

Start in *goat riding* posture with the **Chi Baton™** held at the centre of your chest. (The centre of the **Chi Baton™** should line up with a point in the centre of the sternum on a line between the two nipples. Acupuncture point CV17).

The elbows should be raised, upwards and outwards, as if lifted by two gently inflating balloons, so that they form a line with the *Chi Baton*™. The shoulders should remain relaxed.

On the in breath, **express** as you lift the right arm upwards and across the centre of the body until the *Chi Baton*™ is vertical with the right hand above the left.
Now continue to circle the both arms behind the head until the *Chi Baton*™ is behind the neck. (Be careful to keep your head upright and not to crane your chin forward).

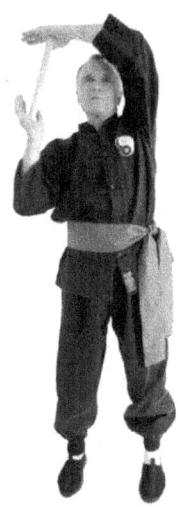

On the out breath, **release** as you lift the left arm over and across the back of the neck until the *Chi Baton*™ is vertical with the left hand above the right.

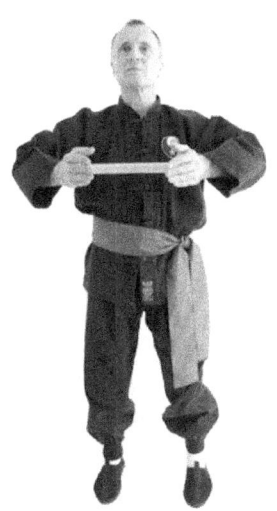

Now continue to circle the left arm forwards until you return to the start position with the *Chi Baton*™ in the centre of your sternum (chest).

Do 6 repetitions in one direction and then reverse the instructions and do 6 repetitions in the opposite direction.

Circle the Moon

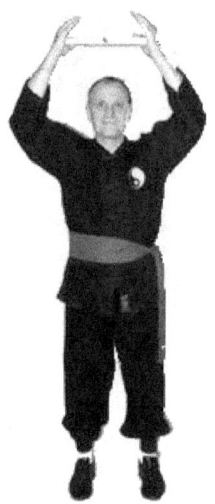

Start in *bear* posture with the **Chi Baton**™ above your head with the elbows relaxed and pointing forwards.

(Keep your shoulders down and relaxed, do not lock your arms, and imagine you are sitting on a "dragon's tail" so that you do not arch your back. Lift your head to look at the baton so that the blood vessels in the neck are not compressed)

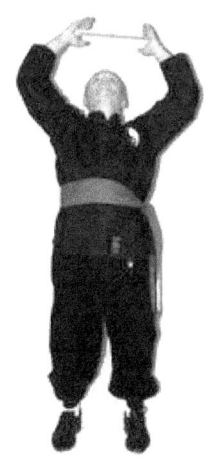

On the in breath, **express** as you circle your upper body backwards, as if drawing a circle on the ceiling. The **Chi Baton**™ stays in the same position relative to the body, and the hips naturally circle to act as a counterbalance. As you circle backwards gently draw your elbows outwards to open up the upper chest.

On the out breath, **release** as you circle your upper body, to bring you back to a forward position. The **Chi**

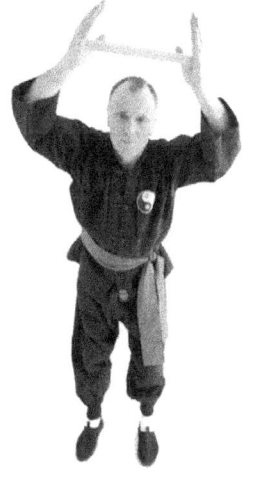

***Baton*™** stays in the same position relative to the body, and the hips again act as a counterbalance. As you rotate forward, relax your elbows, allowing them to draw naturally inward.

Do 6 repetitions in one direction and then reverse the instructions and do 6 repetitions in the other direction.

Avoid the Arrows

(N.B. Hips should remain forward throughout this exercise and knees should not move out of position.)

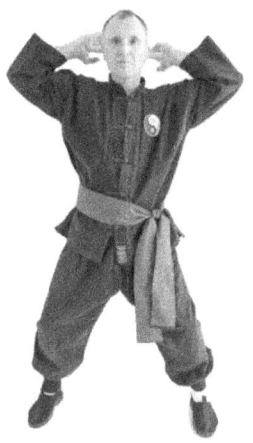

Start in _goat riding_ posture with the **_Chi Baton_**™ behind your neck, and shoulder blades spread.

(Be careful to keep your head upright and not to crane your chin forward).

On the in breath, **express** as you rotate your waist clockwise so that your left elbow is pointing to the front, with the head looking forwards.

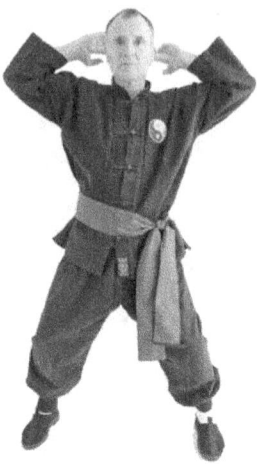

On the out breath, **release,** in a controlled manner, as you unwind, to bring you back to the start position.

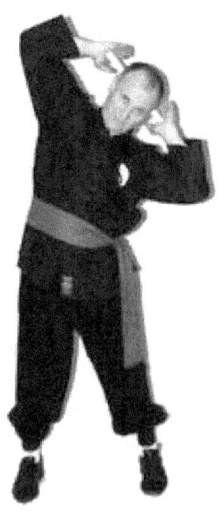

On the in breath, **express** as you extend your right hand side so that your right elbow is pointing to the ceiling, left elbow to the floor, with the head still looking forwards.

(N.B. The right side of the body is <u>extended</u> rather than the left side compressed. Also the weight remains evenly spread between the feet.)

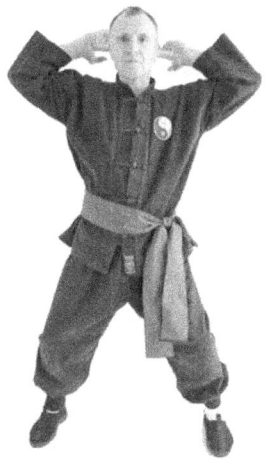

On the out breath, **release,** as you unwind, to bring you back to the start position.

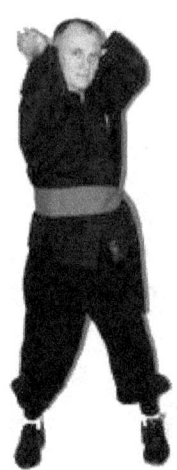

On the in breath, **express** as you rotate your waist anti-clockwise so that your right elbow is pointing to the front, with the head looking forwards.

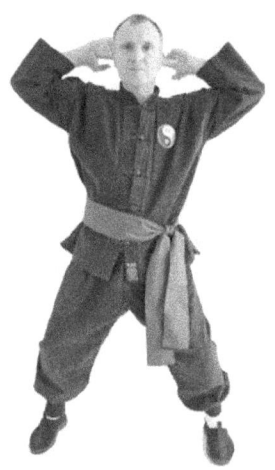

On the out breath, **release,** as you unwind, to bring you back to the start position.

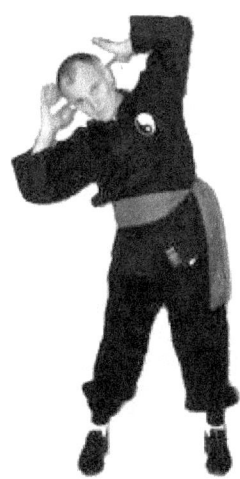

On the in breath, *express* as you extend your left hand side so that your left elbow is pointing to the ceiling, right elbow to the floor, with the head still looking forwards.

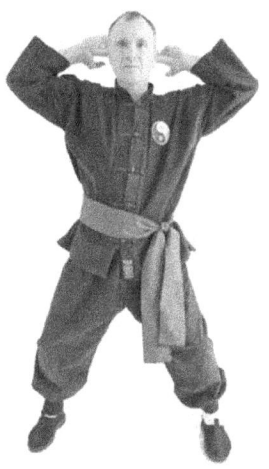

On the out breath, *release,* as you unwind, to bring you back to the start position.

Repeat the movements for another 6 repetitions.

Move the Stones

(N.B. Be careful, in this exercise, not to bend or lock the knees, and keep the weight **evenly** spread between the feet at all times.)

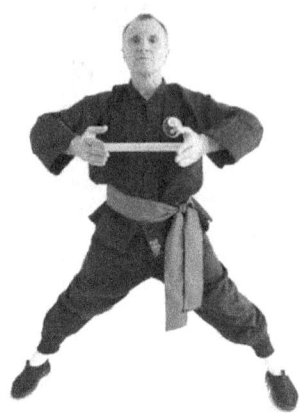

Start in _leg triangle_ posture with the **Chi Baton**™ held at the centre of your chest. The centre of the **Chi Baton**™ should line up with a point in the centre of the sternum on a line between the two nipples. (Acupuncture point CV17).

Breathe in as the elbows are raised,and extended sideways, as if lifted by two gently inflating balloons,so that they form a line with the **Chi Baton**™ . The shoulders should remain relaxed.

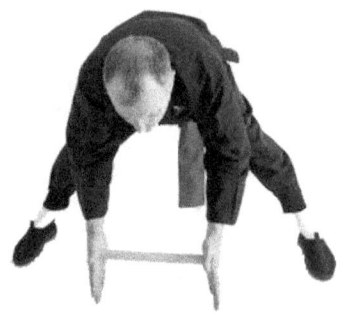

On the out breath, **express** as you bend forward from the hips and slightly extending the arms so that the **Chi Baton**™, is near the floor, as if leaning over a gate. At the same time relax the elbows so that they point down and imagine squeezing energy down the arms.

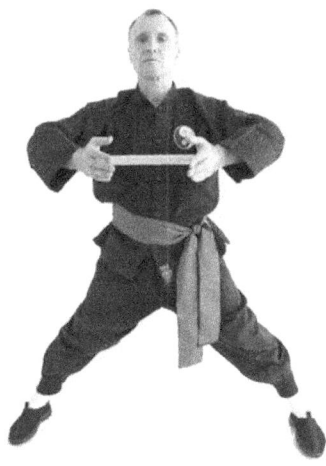

On the in breath, **release,** as you unwind, to bring you back to the start position.

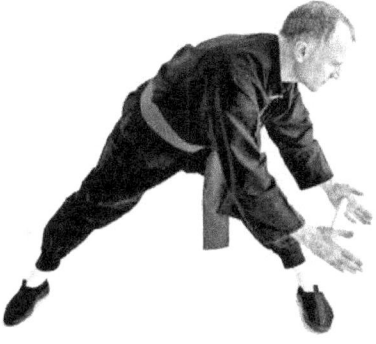

On the out breath, **express** as you turn to the left and bend forward from the hips, slightly extending the arms so that the centre of the **Chi Baton**™ extends down the leg until it is near the floor. At the same time relax the elbows so that they point down and imagine squeezing energy down the arms.

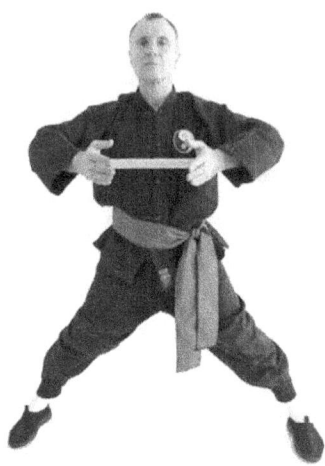

On the in breath, **release,** as you unwind, to bring you back to the start position.

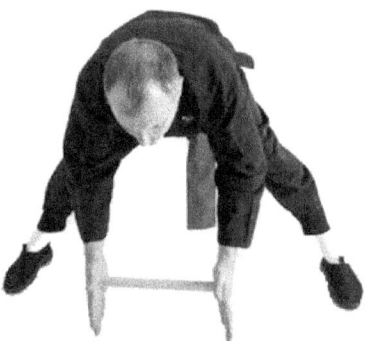

On the out breath, **express** as you bend forward from the hips and slightly extending the arms so that the **Chi Baton**™, is near the floor, as if leaning over a gate. At the same time relax the elbows so that they point down and imagine squeezing energy down the arms.

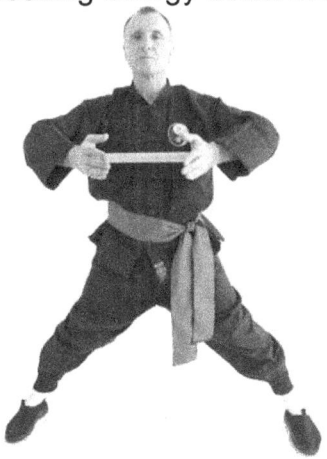

On the in breath, *release,* as you unwind, to bring you back to the start position.

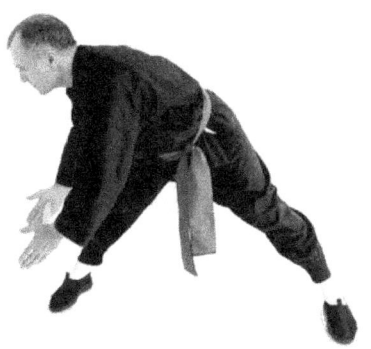

On the out breath, *express* as you turn to the right and bend forward from the hips, slightly extending the arms so that the centre of the *Chi Baton*™ extends down the leg until it is near the floor. At the same time relax the elbows so that they point down and imagine squeezing energy down the arms.

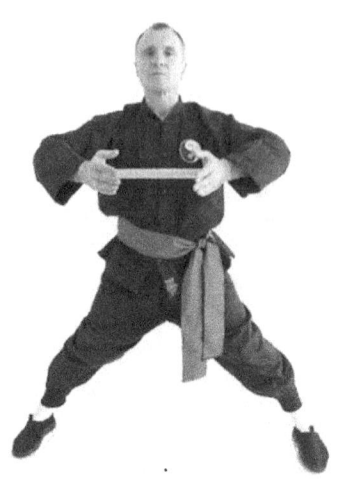

On the in breath, *release,* as you unwind, to bring you back to the start position.

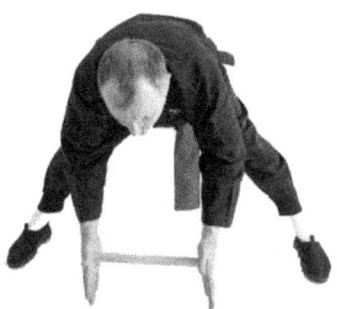

On the out breath, *express* as you bend forward from the hips and slightly extending the arms so that the *Chi Baton*™, is near the floor, as if leaning over a gate. At the same time relax the elbows so that they point down and imagine squeezing energy down the arms.

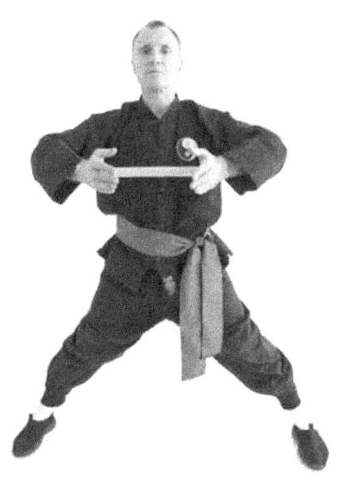

On the in breath, **release,** as you unwind, to bring you back to the start position.

Repeat the movements for another 6 complete repetitions.

Bow to the Emperor

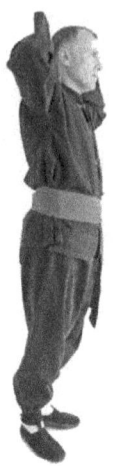

Start in *eagle* posture with the **Chi Baton**™ held behind the neck, ensuring the shoulder blades are spread, and the neck is not craned forward.

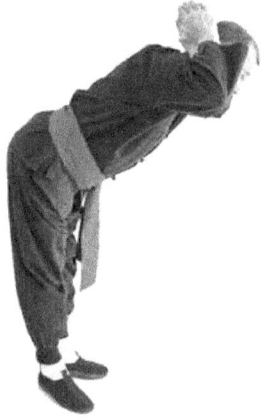

On the out breath, **express,** as you bend forward from the hips, extending through the spine (as if leaning over a gate), until the body is parallel to the floor. (This is a slow movement and should take about five seconds).

On the in breath, release, as you unwind, to bring you back to the start position.

Repeat the movements for another 6 repetitions.

Lift Sky, Press Earth

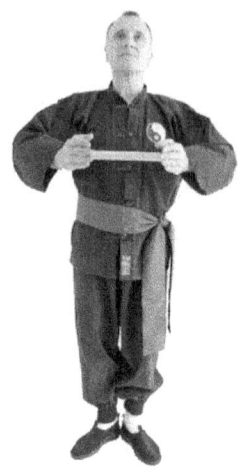

Start in _eagle_ posture with the **_Chi Baton_**™ held in front of the body, at chest height, with elbows forming a straight line with the **_Chi Baton_**™ . (To achieve this, make sure the centre of the **_Chi Baton_**™ is in line with the centre of the sternum, and then imagine two balloons are inflating beneath your elbows to gently lift the elbows upwards and outwards, without raising the shoulders.)

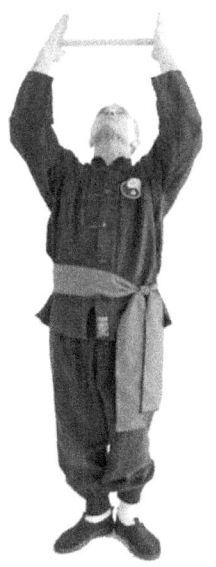

On the out breath, **express,** as you circle the arms forwards and upwards, extending through the spine until the **Chi Baton**™ is above the head. At the same time relax the elbows so that they point forwards. (Remember not to raise the shoulders.)

(As the **Chi Baton**™ passes in front of the face, follow its progress with your eyes, gently lifting the head so that the blood vessels of the neck are not compressed).

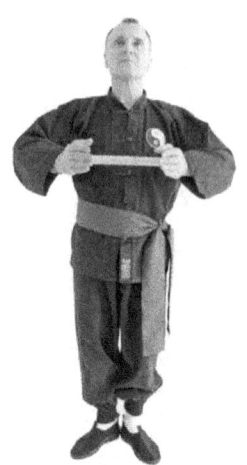

On the in breath, ***release,*** as you unwind, following the same path, to bring you back to the start position.

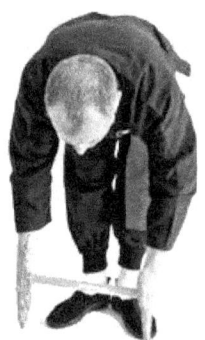

On the out breath, ***express,*** as you extend the spine forwards and outwards from the hips (as if leaning over a gate), relaxing the arms, and head, so that the ***Chi Baton***™ finishes just above the floor.

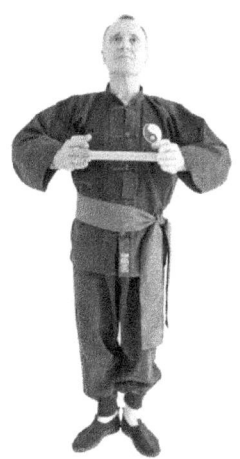

On the in breath, **release,** as you unwind, following the same path, to bring you back to the start position.

Repeat the movements for another 6 repetitions.

Stand Proud

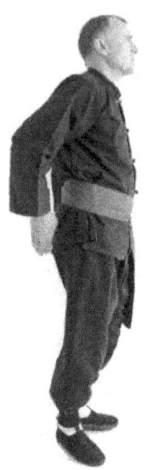

Start in *eagle* posture with the **Chi Baton**™ held behind the body, with relaxed arms down. (In this position, the **Chi Baton**™ is resting against the buttocks.)

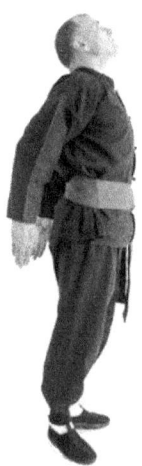

On the in breath, ***express,*** as you tuck the pelvis under, extending the arms downwards, and outwards. At the same, time lift the chest (sternum) and extend the spine strongly upwards.

On the out breath, **release**, to bring you back to the start position.

Repeat the movements for another 6 repetitions.

Release the Arrow

This exercise is performed more slowly than most of the others. (Approximately, 5 seconds per breath.)

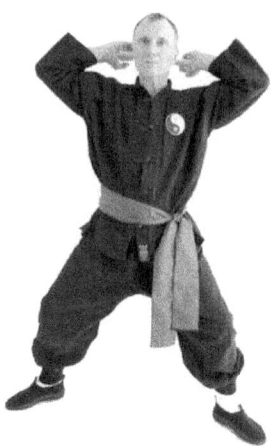

Start in *riding horse* posture, then, turning on the heels, angle the feet outwards 45 degrees. Hold the **Chi Baton**™ behind the neck, being careful not to crane the neck forwards.

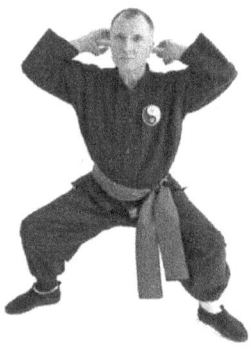

On the out breath, **release,** as you tuck the pelvis under, and squat deeply. Be sure to keep the hip joints open so that the knees stay in line with the feet.

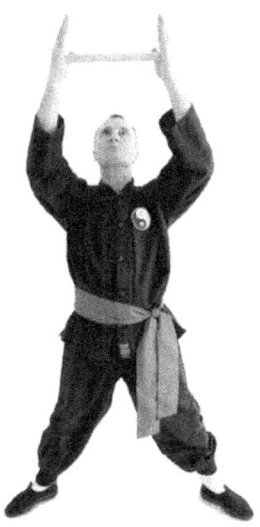

On the in breath, **express**, as you push your pelvis forwards and straighten (but don't lock) the legs. (Be careful not to "bounce" out of the extreme position. You should execute all movements at the same speed, without accelerating or decelerating).

At the same time, extend the **Chi Baton**™ above your head by straightening your arms. (Again, without locking them). Look upwards at the **Chi Baton**™ as you do so, by extending the chin forwards slightly, so that the blood vessel in the neck remain free.

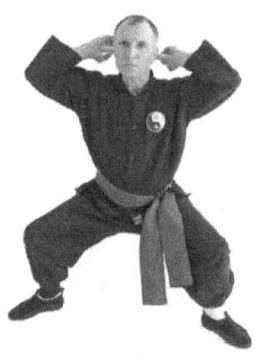

On the out breath, ***release,*** as you tuck the pelvis under, and squat deeply, bringing the ***Chi Baton***™ back to its starting position behind the neck. Remember, as before, to keep the hip joints open so that the knees stay in line with the feet.

Repeat the movements for another 6 repetitions.

Stir the Pot

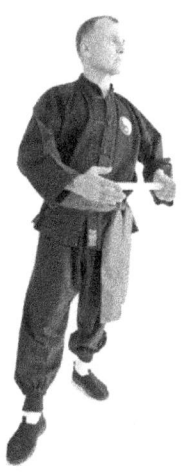

Start in a *duck stance*, (approximately one and a half **Chi Baton**™ distances between your heels), with your left foot forward. Your elbows bend so that your forearms are parallel to the floor. Your upper body is slightly turned to the left with your hips forward.

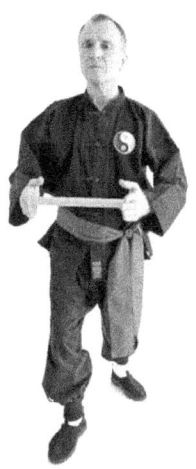

On the out breath, **express,** as you rotate your waist anti-clockwise, and transfer your weight forwards into a *dragon stance.* The **Chi Baton**™ should circle in the same direction as the waist. It is important that the arms hardly lengthen at all, and stay in the same place relative to the body. The circle happens because the waist is circling. Be careful to keep the knees pointing along the line of the toes to prevent straining the knees. The whole action is with the waist.

On the in breath, **release**, as you lift your belly and continue the anti-clockwise circle to bring you back to the start position.

Repeat the movements for another 6 repetitions, then change legs and perform the exercise in the opposite direction.

Repulse the Demons

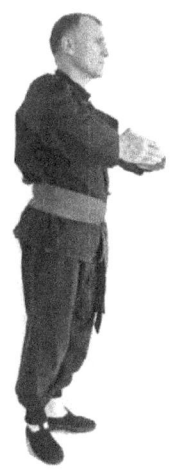

Start in _eagle stance_, **Chi Baton**™ held in line with the centre of your chest, elbows in line with the **Chi Baton**™ with your shoulders relaxed.

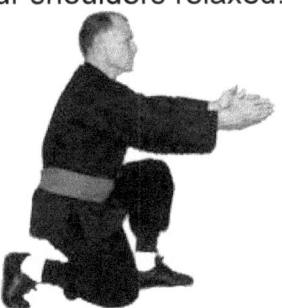

On the out breath, **express,** as you step forward one **Chi Baton**™ pace, smartly, with your left foot, raising your right heel and sinking downwards. You should finish in _chicken stance,_ with your right knee just above the ground, and slightly behind the front heel. <u>Do not push the left knee over the line of the front toes, or</u>

incline the body too far forwards as this will over strain the front knee.

At the same time, relax the elbows and extend your arms forward.

On the out breath, **release**, as you steadily push off your left leg, lift your body upwards and step back into the starting position. The arms draw back inwards and the elbows gently rise as if lifted by gently inflating balloons so that they are in line with the baton.

Repeat the movements for another 6 repetitions, then change legs and perform the exercise in the opposite direction.

Row the Boat

(On the next three exercises, when leaning back the heels will naturally draw towards you slightly, and extend slightly on the forward movement. This action prevents straining the lower spine so be careful not to wear shoes that "stick" and prevent this natural movement.

Sit in double plough stance, with spine upright and legs relaxed and slightly "off lock". The toes should be pointing upright, with feet, knees and ankles in a straight line (Approximately one *Chi Baton*™ distance apart from middle toe to middle toe). The *Chi Baton*™ is held in the usual position in front of the chest with the arms raised about two fist distances from the body.

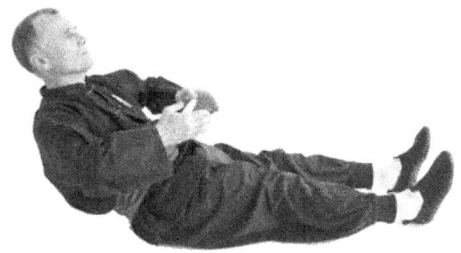

As you breath in, lean back 45 degrees.

At the same time bring the centre of the *Chi Baton*™ to the centre of your chest.

The *Chi Baton*™ should be at least two fist distances from your chest, and the elbows should be gently raised upwards and outwards, as if lifted by balloons. This ensures that the upper chest is open to facilitate easy breathing.

81

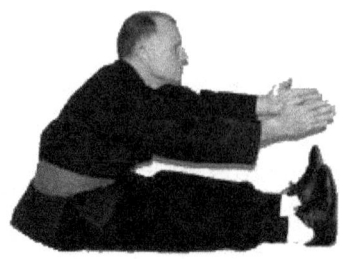

As you breath out, **express,** bringing your body forwards, by bending from the hips, expanding the spine, relaxing the elbows, and slightly extending your arms.

The **Chi Baton**™ should remain at the same height relative to the floor, as if you are sliding it along a table.

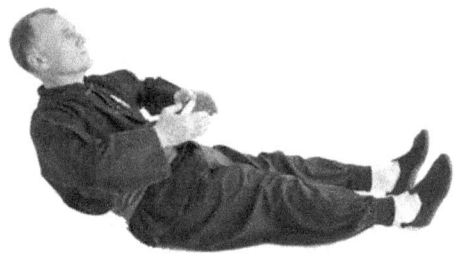

On the next in breath **release** as you return to the start position, with the body angled at 45 degrees and the elbows raised etc.

Do six repetitions.

(N.B. Be disciplined in remembering to raise the elbows! It is all to easy to let them droop after a few movements. Raising the elbows each in breath gives a workout to the upper body as well as ensuring correct respiration.)

Brush the Foot

Sit in double plough stance, as for the previous exercise, with spine upright and legs relaxed and slightly "off lock". The toes should be pointing upright, with feet, knees and ankles in a straight line.

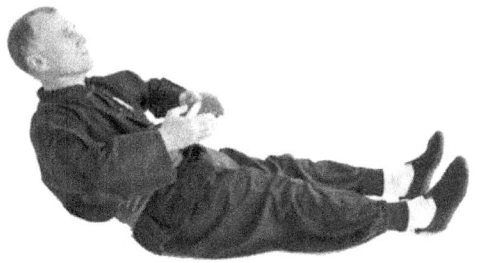

As you breath in, lean back 45 degrees.

At the same time bring the centre of the *Chi Baton*™ to the centre of your chest.

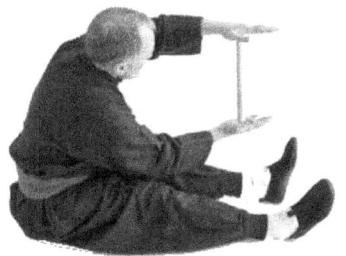

As you breath out, *express,* bringing your body forwards by expanding the spine, relaxing the elbows, and slightly extending your arms.

At the same time, twist through the axis of the spine so that the *Chi Baton*™ finishes vertical, over the left foot, with the left hand above the right.

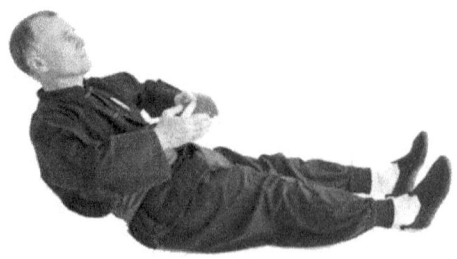

On the next in breath *release* as you return to the start position with the body angled at 45 degrees and the elbows raised etc.

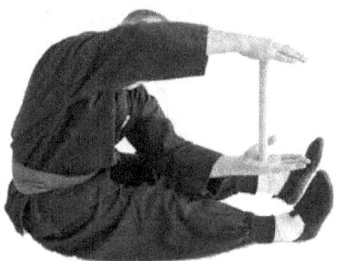

As you breath out, *express,* bringing your body forwards by expanding the spine and slightly extending your arms.

At the same time, twist through the axis of the spine so that the *Chi Baton*™ finishes vertical, over the right foot, with the right hand above the left.

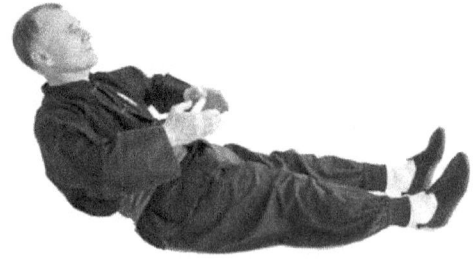

On the next in breath *release* as you return to the start position with the body angled at 45 degrees and the elbows raised etc.

Do six repetitions.

(N.B. Be disciplined in remembering to raise the elbows! It is all to easy to let them droop after a few movements. Raising the elbows each in breath gives a workout to the upper body as well as ensuring correct respiration.)

Work the Shuttles

Sit in double plough stance, with spine upright and legs relaxed and slightly "off lock". The toes should be pointing upright, with feet, knees and ankles in a straight line.

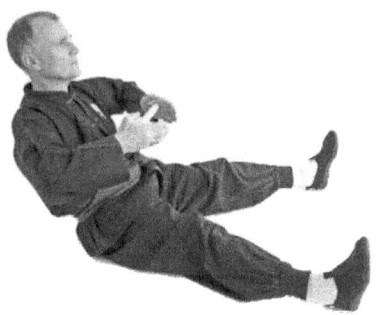

As you breath in, lean back 45 degrees, and open your legs as wide as you comfortably can.

At the same time bring the centre of the **Chi Baton**™ to the centre of your chest, in its usual position.

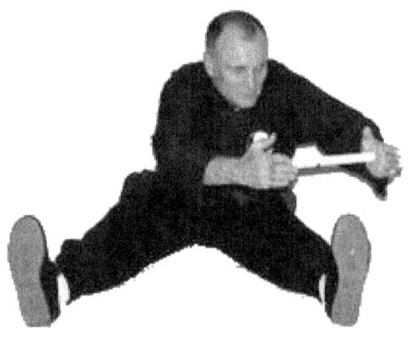

As you breath out, ***express,*** twisting the body to the left and, by bending from the hips, extend down the left leg, expanding the spine and slightly extending your arms.

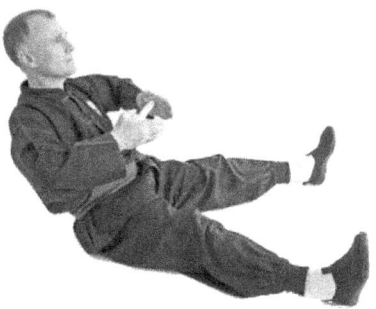

On the next in breath *release* as you return to the start position with the body angled at 45 degrees and the elbows raised etc.

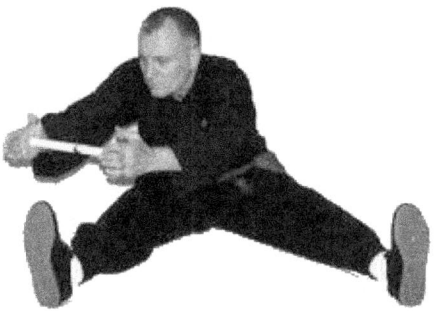

As you breath out, *express,* twisting the body to the right and extending down the right leg by bending from the hips, expanding the spine and slightly extending your arms.

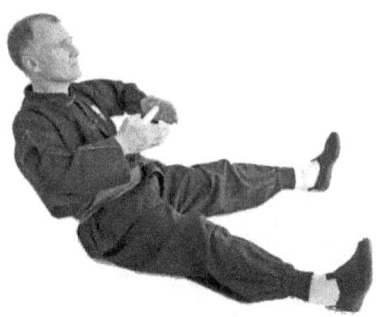

On the next in breath *release* as you return to the start position with the body angled at 45 degrees and the elbows raised etc.

Do six repetitions.

(N.B. Be disciplined in remembering to raise the elbows! It is all to easy to let them droop after a few movements. Raising the elbows each in breath gives a workout to the upper body as well as ensuring correct respiration.)

Walk the Hills

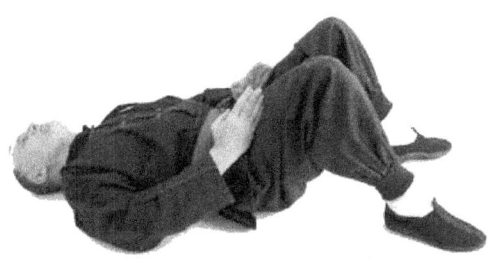

Lie on your back with your knees drawn up in a comfortable position, with the **Chi Baton**™ resting on your lap.

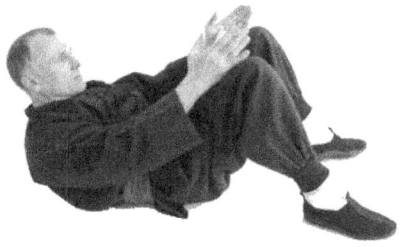

As you breath out, **express,** curling the body, expanding the spine and slightly extending your arms, so that the edges of the hands holding the **Chi Baton**™ slide up your thighs. (Imagine you are holding a tennis ball under your chin as you do so to prevent cramping the neck). This is a slow movement and should take at least five seconds.

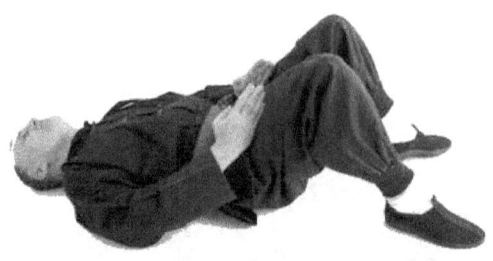

On the next in breath **release**, in a controlled manner, and slowly roll the spine back to return to the start position.

Do six repetitions.

Cat Stretches

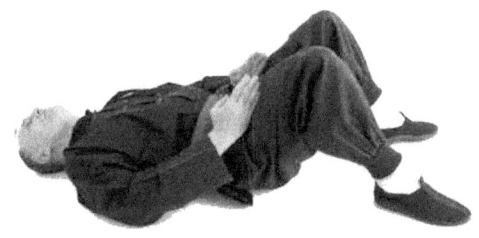

Lie on your back with your knees drawn up in a comfortable position, with the *Chi Baton*™ resting on your lap.

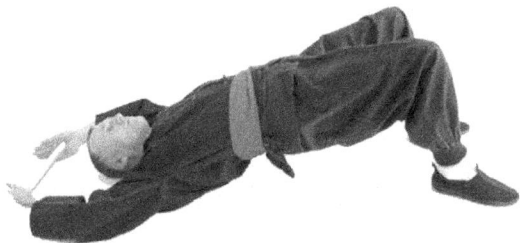

As you breath in, *express,* curling the pelvis under, to roll and lift the pelvis and the spine off the ground. At the same time circle the arms above the head so that the *Chi Baton*™ rests on the floor. At the end of the move, draw the elbows outwards, and back slightly, to open up the sides of the chest.

On the out breath, *release,* in a controlled manner, and slowly return to the start position, trying to ensure that each vertebra touches the floor as you do so.

Do six repetitions.

(Reminder: Remember each movement is a controlled four seconds)

Knee Drops

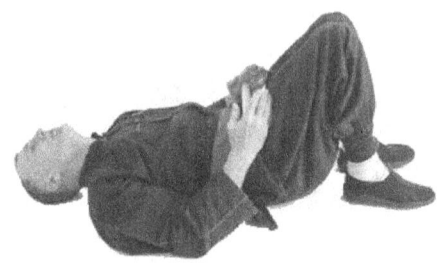

Lie on your back with your knees drawn up as close to the buttocks as possible, with the **Chi Baton**™ resting on your lap.

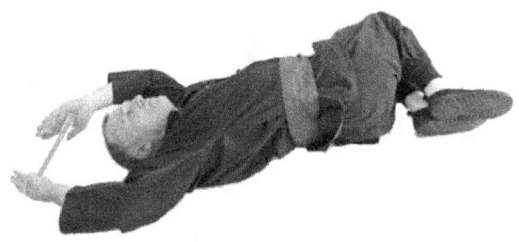

As you breath in, **express,** as you take both knees to the left hand side, aiming to touch the ground if possible, but without allowing your shoulders to lift off the floor.

At the same time circle the arms above the head so that the **Chi Baton**™ rests on the floor. At the end of the move, spread the elbows outwards, to open up the sides of the chest.

On the out breath, **release,** reverse the movement, and slowly return to the start position.

Repeat the movement to the other side to complete the

sequence.

Do another repetition both sides.

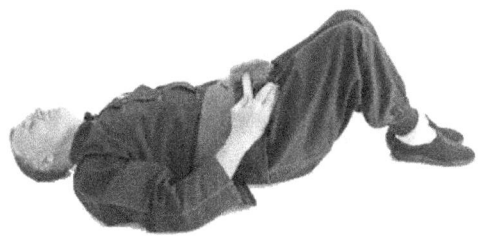

Slide your feet away from you so that they are now where your knees would be if your legs were straight, with the **Chi Baton**™ resting on your lap.

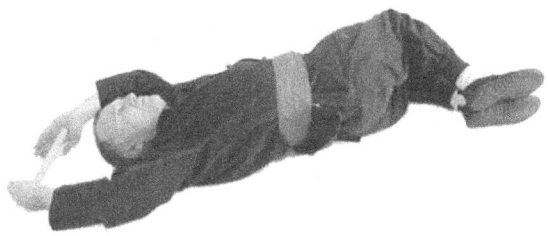

As you breath in, **express,** as you take both knees to the left hand side, aiming to touch the ground if possible, but without allowing your shoulders to lift off the floor.

At the same time circle the arms above the head so that the **Chi Baton**™ rests on the floor. At the end of the move, draw the elbows outwards, and back slightly, to open up the sides of the chest.

On the out breath, **release,** reverse the movement, and slowly return to the start position.

Repeat the movement to the other side to complete the

sequence.

Do another repetition both sides.

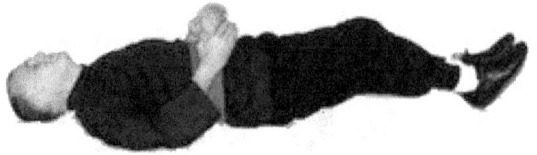

Slide your feet away from you so that they are now where your ankles would be if your legs were straight, (the feet will be slightly angled upwards in this position), with the **Chi Baton**™ resting on your lap.

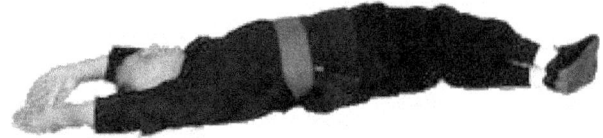

As you breath in, **express,** as you take both knees to the left hand side, aiming to touch the ground if possible, but without allowing your shoulders to lift off the floor.

At the same time circle the arms above the head so that the **Chi Baton**™ rests on the floor. At the end of the move, draw the elbows outwards, and back slightly, to open up the sides of the chest.

On the out breath, **release,** reverse the movement, and slowly return to the start position.

Repeat the movement to the other side to complete the sequence.

Do another repetition, both sides.

Forward Leg Raises

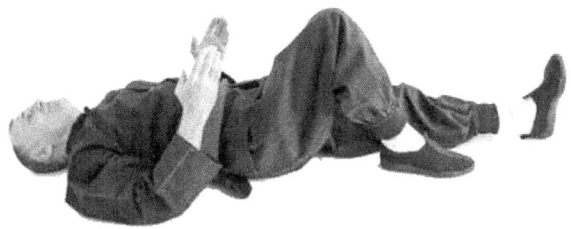

Lie on your back with your right knee drawn up in a comfortable position. The left leg is straight, without locking the knee joint, with the foot pointing to the ceiling. The *Chi Baton*™ rests on your lap.

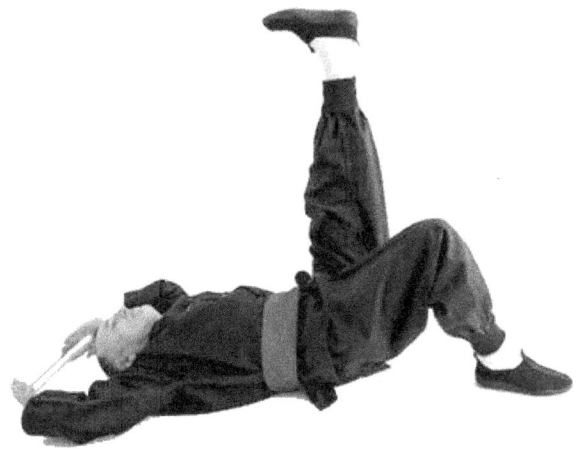

As you breath in, **express,** as you extend through the heel, curl the pelvis under, and lift the left leg as high as possible, without straining. Keep the leg as straight as possible without locking the knee. (As you become stronger, you may wish to supplement this action by pushing down on the supporting leg.)

At the same time circle the arms above the head so that

the **Chi Baton**™ rests on the floor. At the end of the move, draw the elbows outwards, and back slightly, to open up the sides of the chest.

On the out breath, **release,** and slowly return to the start position, in a controlled manner.

Do six repetitions.
Repeat the movements to the other side to complete the sequence.

Side Leg Raises

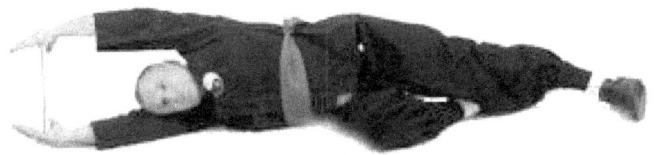

Lie on your right hand side with your right knee drawn up/forwards in a comfortable position, supporting your weight, so that the heel is in line with the buttock. (This helps to keep the pelvis tilted under slightly and helps prevent back strain.)

The left leg is straight, without locking the knee joint. The arms holding the **Chi Baton**™ are straight, but not locked, above the head, and the head is resting on your right arm. (This helps to ensure that the spine is kept as straight as possible without strain).

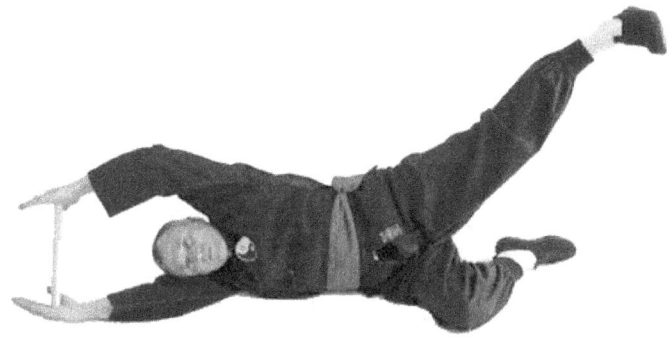

As you breath in, **express,** as you extend through the heel, and lift the left leg vertically, as high as possible, without straining. The foot remains parallel to the floor to ensure the correct motion of the hip joint. (As you become stronger, you may wish to supplement this action by pushing down on the right leg.)

On the out breath, **release,** and slowly return to the start position.

Do six repetitions.

Repeat the movements to the other side to complete the sequence.

Rear Leg Raises

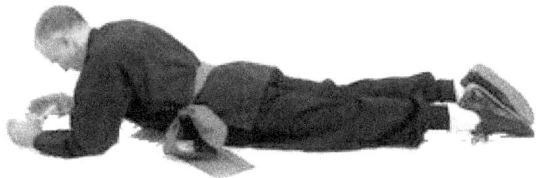

Lie, face down, in a comfortable position, supporting your weight on your forearms, which are holding the *Chi Baton*™.

Your upper body is raised in a *Cobra* position, with the head relaxed down.

The legs are relaxed, with the two bones at the front of the pelvis resting on the floor. These two bones remain in contact with the floor throughout this exercise. This ensures that the back is not over strained.

The legs are kept straight throughout, without locking the knee joints of course.

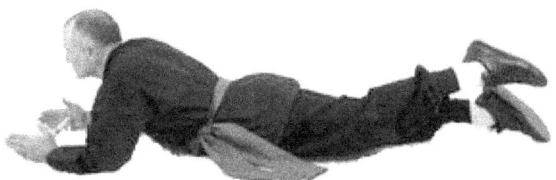

As you breath in, ***express,*** as you extend through the **toe**, and lift the left leg vertically, as high as possible, without straining. (Remember to keep the two bones at the front of the pelvis resting on the floor) At the same time extend your chin forwards, without compressing the back of the neck.

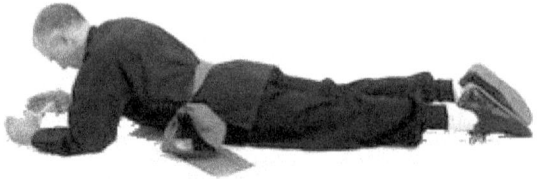

On the out breath, *release,* and slowly return to the start position.

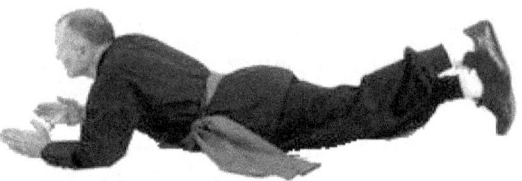

As you breath in, *express,* as you extend through the **heel** this time, and lift the same left leg vertically, as high as possible, without straining. (Again, remember to keep the two bones at the front of the pelvis resting on the floor.) At the same time extend your chin forwards.

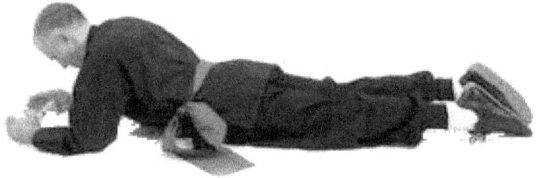

On the out breath, *release,* and slowly return to the start position.

Do six repetitions (alternating between pointing the toe and expressing through the heel).

Repeat the movements to the other side to complete the sequence.

(N.B. This exercise is more effective if you do not rest your leg, on the floor between repetitions.)

Crocodile

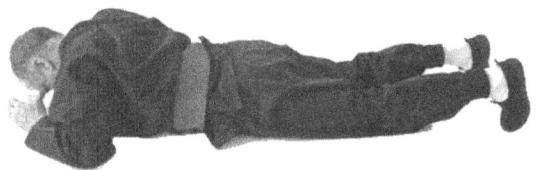

Lie, face down, in a comfortable position, with your forehead resting on the *Chi Baton*™, and the toes drawn under.

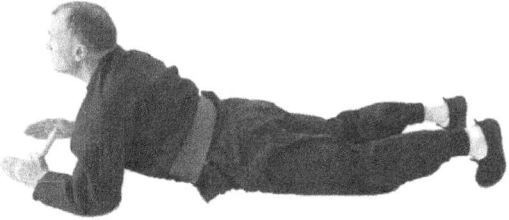

As you breath in, *express,* and raise the upper body into a *Cobra* position.

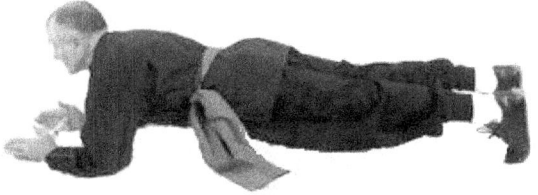

On the out breath, **continue to *express,*** and slowly lift your hips so that the body is parallel to the floor, supported by your forearms and the tips of you toes.

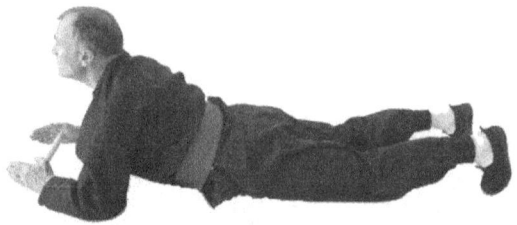

As you breath in, ***release,*** and lower the hips back into the *Cobra* position again.

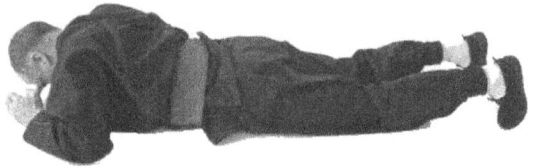

As you breath out, **continue to *release,*** and lower the upper body into a comfortable position with your forehead resting on the ***Chi Baton*™**.

Do six repetitions

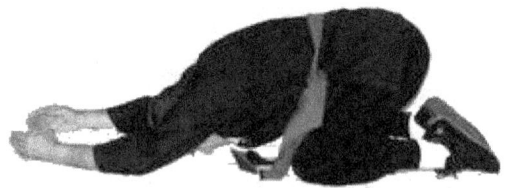

N.B. On completion of this exercise, with the arms still resting on the floor, sit back on to your heels, relax and stretch the back out again for a couple of minutes before continuing.

Stand Still (Close).

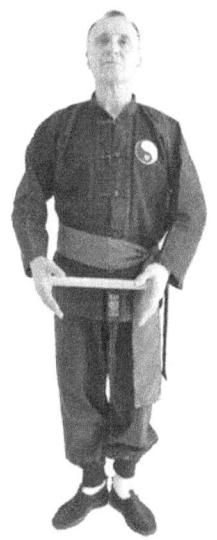

Stand in *Bear Stance,* holding the rod at stomach height, with the shoulders and elbows relaxed. Keep the tongue on the roof of the mouth and focus on circulating energy from the stomach, across the **Chi Baton**™ , back to the stomach making a triangle of energy. Do this for about a minute to ensure that all your energy is correctly in place.

Chi Cutout

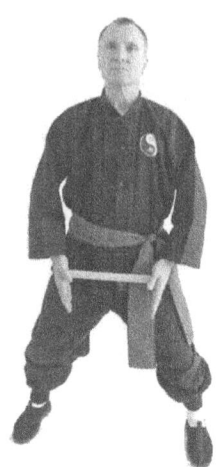

Stand in *Riding Horse*, holding the **Chi Baton**™ with the arms relaxed and the fingers pointing down.

As you breath in to the chest, ***express***, and focus on drawing energy upwards to fill the upper chest. (Imagine you are drawing energy up through your feet.) Slightly draw the elbows outwards as you breathe in.

As you breath out, ***release***.

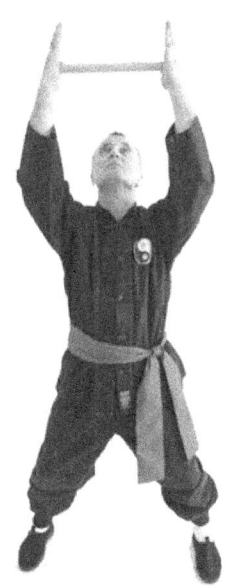

As you breath in to the belly, **express**, and lift your arms up so that the fingers are pointing to the ceiling, with the elbows forwards. Follow the movement of the **Chi Baton**™ with your eyes so that you end up looking upwards. Focus on drawing energy downwards to fill the belly. (Imagine you are drawing energy down through the top of your head.)

As you breath out, **release.**

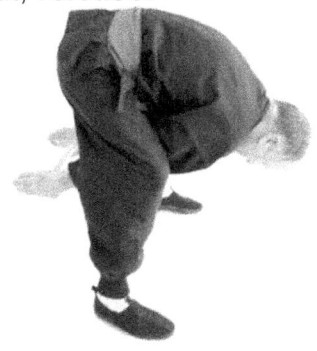

As you breath in, **express**, as you bend forwards from the hips, and take the **Chi Baton**™ as far between your legs as you comfortably can. Hold your breath in this position for five seconds.

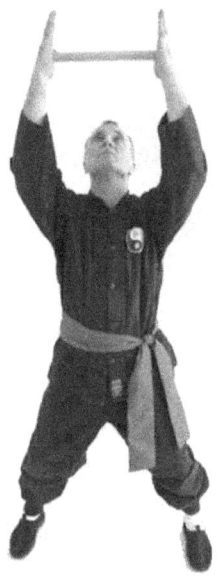

As you breath out, **release**, and return to the hands above the head position.

As you breath in to the belly, **express**, and focus on drawing energy down. (Imagine you are drawing energy down through the top of your head.)

As you breath out, **release**.

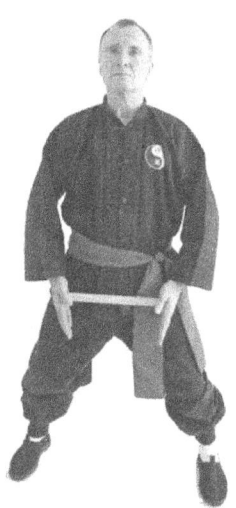

As you breath in to the chest, **express**, and gently lower the arms down to the fingers down position. and focus on drawing energy upwards. (Imagine you are drawing energy up through your feet.)

As you breath out, **release**, and allow any excess energy to flow away out of your body.

This exercise is only performed once.

Relax and enjoy the glow of energy as it travels around the body.

If you enjoyed this book, you may like to know that other **Chi Baton™**, publications, by **Barry Westley**, will be out shortly. Each of the further publications will follow a similar format to this book, but will have a different blend of exercises that highlight different aspects of the **Chi Baton™ Exercise System.**

In the pipeline are further **Chi Baton™** Manuals, plus a **Chi Baton™ Manual of Seated Exercises**. (This contains all the principles of normal **Chi Baton™** exercises, but is suitable for those with severe arthritis or limited mobility, as well as able bodied students).

To compliment the books, a series of DVD's of **Barry Westley,** performing the various programmes, will also be produced.

For more information,
Web: www.chibaton.co.uk)

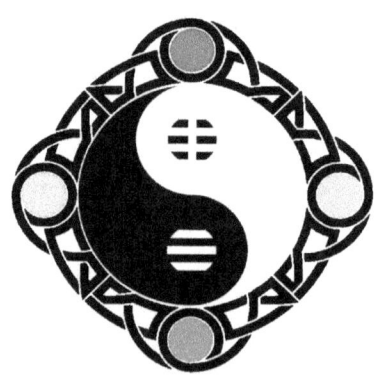

Barry Westley 2014 ©